# Chronic Progressive

# Marion Deutsche Cohen

Plain View Press
P. O. 42255
Austin, TX 78704

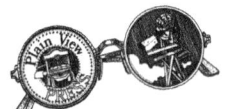

plainviewpress.net
sb@plainviewpress.net
512-441-2452

Copyright Marion Deutsche Cohen, 2009. All rights reserved.
ISBN: 978-1-935514-23-7
Library of Congress Number: 2009929323

## Acknowledgements

Some of these poems have appeared in: *Facets, Mainstay* (the well spouse newsletter), *Minetta, Trillium, Schuykill Valley Poets, Palo Alto Review, Bridges Art/Math* conference proceedings, *Take Care!* (the newsletter of the National Family Caregivers Association), *Extreme Points* (chapbook, Center for Thanatology Research), *"Ex-spouses of Deceased Spouses"* anthology, *Slow Dancing to Invisible Music* (2007 anthology; *"Progressive #5"* won honorable mention in that anthology.), *Lob der Funfeck (Praise for Pentagons,* an anthology of mathematical poetry; *"A Mathematician in the Family"* was translated into German.), *The Eloquent Atheist, "Surviving the Alphabet"* (chapbook, Huge Pathetic Force Press, PA)

Cover art: by Devin Asher Cohen

## Other Books By Marion Deutsche Cohen

Poetry: *Tuesday Nights (ed. with Wemara Dare), The Weirdest Is the Sphere, She Was Born She Died, Mother-Poet (ed.), The Limits of Miracles (ed.), Counting to Zero: poems on repeated miscarriage, The Sitting-Down Hug, These Covers to Crawl Under, The Level of Doorknobs, The Temper Tantrum Book, Extreme Points, Epsilon Country, Crossing the Equal Sign, and Surviving the Alphabet*

Non-fiction: *An Ambitious Sort of Grief: Diary of Neonatal Loss, The Shadow of an Angel: Diary of Subsequent Pregnancy, A Garden Flower: Diary of Cesarean Birth and Life with the Subsequent Baby, The Level of Doorknobs, and Dirty Details: The Days and Nights of a Well Spouse*

*to my children Marielle, Arin, Bret, and Devin, who struggled with (and sometimes without) me -- and to Jon, who was cool enough to join us*

# Contents

# Part I: Wrought With Efficiency

| | |
|---|---|
| Bach Magnificat | 15 |
| Self Portrait With Catheter Bag | 16 |
| Progressive #5 | 17 |
| End Stage | 18 |
| Catheter Bag Tubing | 19 |
| "Thrift Store Paradise" | 20 |
| The Ocean | 21 |
| Of Dresses, Colors, and 3:48 A.M. | 22 |
| Self Portrait With Catheter Bag #2 | 24 |
| He Sleeps Raised | 25 |
| Untitled | 26 |
| Temper Tantrum For That Taxi Driver | 27 |
| Writing As a Disability | 28 |
| Demonstration: April 30, 1992 | 29 |
| Bathroom Rumpus Again | 30 |
| Notes On Sleep Deprivation | 31 |
| Summer Exacerbations | 32 |
| Summer Of '92 | 33 |
| Questions, 1993 | 35 |
| Progressive '93 | 36 |
| More Notes On Sleep Deprivation | 37 |
| Last Night's 2:00 A.M. | 38 |
| Rehab | 39 |
| Reasons To Cry | 40 |
| The Back Up Poem | 41 |
| Thirty-Five Years | 42 |
| This Is a Home | 43 |
| Training New Aides: One Thing I'm Tired Of | 44 |
| This Is a House | 45 |
| Self-Portrait With Catheter Bag #3 | 46 |

| | |
|---|---|
| Significant Adolescent Dream | 47 |
| Goofing Off As a Disability | 48 |
| Ode To Able-Bodied-Ness | 49 |
| Bedroom, Midnight | 51 |
| Progressive, Progressive, Progressive | 52 |
| Notes On Being Tired In General | 55 |
| Despair | 56 |
| On the Train | 57 |

## Part II: Out Of the Frying Pan

| | |
|---|---|
| The First Nursing Home Dream | 61 |
| The First Nursing Home Reality | 62 |
| Not Grieving | 63 |
| Sick | 64 |
| Sick #2 | 65 |
| Weepy These Days | 66 |
| Welcoming Address To the Nursing Home Staff | 67 |
| The End Of That Dream | 68 |
| Friend | 69 |
| At His Mouth | 70 |
| Following Him Into the MRI | 71 |
| About Sex | 72 |
| On the Toilet, Me | 73 |
| Notes On a Current Pet Peeve | 74 |
| Dream In Which I Was Only Talking | 75 |
| On the Need To Be Heard | 76 |
| Dream Of the Dinner For Two | 77 |
| Where Loneliness Begins | 78 |
| Contemplating the Second Time Around | 79 |
| After a Bad Evening a Mean Little Voice Tries To Whip Me Into Shape | 80 |
| The Fury Of the Living | 81 |
| Reading A Book This Particular Day | 82 |

| | |
|---|---|
| The Misfortune Cookie #2 | 83 |
| Christmas 1993 | 84 |
| August 3,1993 | 85 |
| The Last Love Poem For Jeff | 86 |
| Progressive #Umpteen | 87 |
| March 6, 1998 | 89 |
| Wanting To Rhyme | 90 |
| Courtship Memory | 92 |
| Especially Progressive That Day | 93 |
| On Reading To Sick People | 94 |
| Where I Stand These Days | 95 |
| Signs Of Dementia | 96 |
| The Beginning Of Being Dead | 97 |
| On Movies vs. Plays | 98 |
| Chronic | 99 |
| A Writer's Little Nightmare | 100 |
| Thinking About the Second Time Around | 101 |
| The Life and Habits Of the Well Spouse | 102 |
| Deciding Against the Second Time Around | 103 |
| But the Dermatologist | 104 |
| A Mathematician In the Family | 105 |
| The Second Time Around, More Thoughts and Fears | 106 |
| More About Lips | 107 |
| A New Vow | 108 |
| Wanting Him To Die | 110 |
| Alone | 111 |
| January 2001 | 112 |
| Online Personal Ads As a Disability | 113 |
| Untitled | 114 |
| Personals 101 (a series of limericks) | 115 |
| September 11 and the Single Woman | 117 |
| Hurt | 118 |
| March 22, 2002 | 119 |
| Another No | 120 |
| The Problem | 121 |

| | |
|---|---:|
| Monday Morning, Unemployed | 122 |
| Perish | 123 |
| The Imposter | 124 |
| Conversation With the Mirror | 125 |
| Self In 2001 | 126 |
| How I Know I'm Still Alive | 128 |
| How I Know This Is a Dream | 129 |
| How I Know About the Law Of Averages | 130 |
| Parable Of the Life-Affirming Woman | 131 |
| A Short Song Of Agony | 132 |
| Short Agony #2 | 133 |
| Slowly | 134 |
| A Bad Week | 135 |
| Another Misfortune Cookie | 136 |
| Murphy's Laws Of Probability, 2001 | 137 |
| Cochlear | 138 |
| Roses | 139 |
| What's Theoretically Possible | 140 |
| Honorary | 141 |
| Cancer Scare | 142 |
| Mozart To The Gills | 143 |
| The Beginning Of Courage | 144 |
| Diarist's Strike | 145 |
| Another Helpful Metaphor | 146 |
| I Disguise My House | 147 |
| "Memento" | 148 |
| The Revolt Of the Chosen | 149 |

## Part III: Out Of the Fire

| | |
|---|---:|
| Falling In Love | 153 |
| Songs For the Good New Year | 154 |
| Lips and Pants | 155 |
| Dream Of Hanky Panky | 156 |

| | |
|---|---|
| My New Love In the Early Morning | 157 |
| A Quiet Man | 158 |
| Dream Of Someone Dying | 159 |
| Progressive Becomes Progress | 160 |
| One Woman Show | 162 |
| The Jeff Complex | 163 |
| Instead Of Dying | 164 |
| This Versus It | 165 |
| Death Still Takes a Holiday | 166 |
| Like a False Pregnancy | 167 |
| One Line Untitled | 168 |
| Phone Call From the Hospital A La Molly Bloom | 169 |
| On Getting Engaged the Day After My Husband Dies | 171 |
| Calling a Spade a Spade | 172 |
| Love Poem For a New Love | 173 |
| Wedding Preparations Former Well Spouse Style | 175 |
| Wedding Vows | 176 |
| Impossible Dreams | 177 |
| Post | 178 |
| Dream That Jon Acquires a Wheelchair | 179 |
| The Human Spirit | 180 |
| Dream Of Easier Changes | 182 |
| Possibilities | 183 |
| Notes | 185 |
| About the Author | 191 |

# Part I: Wrought With Efficiency

## Bach Magnificat

These infested pages, armies of eighth notes, bearing and
    thrusting those long thick spears, not one rest, not one
    truce. "Take short breaths at the commas," she says.
Little mini-gasps, half-unit dreams at the commas in the text
and there are indeed commas, there are commas aplenty,
    the text is peaceful, the text is kind.
But maybe I'll make a mistake and breathe out instead of in,
maybe I'll breathe *all* the way out, or breathe in but too far,
    irretrievable, or retrieve too much, too much too soon.
Even done just right these epsilon breaths don't feel like
    breaths, don't feel like anything, my lungs are rigid, my
    lungs are numb. I'm not suffocating, I don't need air but I
    want air, I want it bad, want to feel the air, want to feel it
    go in.
Like Jeff at night, a close July night, he'd wake up and try to
    feel himself breathe but the air'd be lukewarm, too warm
    to feel; he'd be getting it, I'd see his chest getting it but
    he couldn't feel it, couldn't know it, couldn't collect it and
    from sleep he'd mumble and grope, from sleep he'd panic
    but good.
And like now, on the respirator, he definitely gets the air, he
    has to get the air but, like the kids say, he doesn't do it, he
    doesn't feel himself doing it, he gets done, gets breathed.
The kids don't like that, fifteen breaths per minute no matter
    what, page after page of four- second breaths
not one eighth-note, not one rest.

## Self Portrait With Catheter Bag

Her legs are bent. Her head is straight.
She is looking all around.
She seems to be actually posing for a portrait
and she seems to not quite know
what the artist will make of her.
She could be waiting for a bus.
She could be waiting for a friend.
She could be working on a puzzle.
She could be working out a knot.
Or she could be a wallflower
at the high-school dance.
Her hands are very busy.
Her feet are very still.

## Progressive #5

He can still hold the jar
I position his hands
can still sit up
I position his feet
can still lie down
I position his head
still make love
I position his position.
He knows the place
but keeps asking the time
and what's for supper
and where are the cats?
And around seven
what movies we have
and are they funny?
he wants them funny
if they're not funny
he needs his head scratched.
He keeps renewing
old regrets
and keeps creating
new regrets.
His old regrets
feel new.
His new regrets
feel old.

## End Stage

He lies stiff.
Not dead but stiff.
Chronically, progressively, incurably stiff.
Range of motion on his left arm takes a minute.
Range of motion on his right arm takes five minutes.
"Bend me forward." "Move my legs apart." "Scratch the right
 side of my nose."
There is no point in saying please.

He is not yet bed-ridden.
Only chair-ridden.
But he's in bed right now.
And it's not bedtime.

Paralyzed means stiff.
Paralyzed means locked.
Paralyzed means *we*
can't move him, either.

## Catheter Bag Tubing

In the morning it acquires a life of its own. The snake inside it
   uncoils. We find it out of its square, sniffing around, shak-
   ingly testing the floor.
Later, in the bathroom, I try to put both ends simultaneously
   where they belong,
I hold the top end but the bottom end dives, I catch it
   sneaking out the bowl and, even before the escape, it curls
   up and away.

And then the final spreading, the ultimate sweeping
like a child
like a searchlight
like outstretched arms.

## "Thrift Store Paradise"

*(name of a thrifting workshop I once facilitated)*

These arms and legs
are only clothes.
They have no head.
They have no toes.
No mouth to feed.
No teeth to brush.
No motion to range.
No spasm to hush.
Nose won't itch.
Mouth won't spit.
Crotch won't pee.
Butt won't shit.
These clothes are so clean.
These clothes are so light.
And they don't wake up
all hours of the night.
So face your partners.
Bow and smile.
And promenade them
down the aisle.
Yes, face your partners
and a do-si-do's.
For they're only clothes.
Only clothes.

## The Ocean

I went in up to my neck, beyond the breakers
nothing was broken, not even a crack
it all lay flat, too smooth and flat.
I stood there and turned, and then turned back.
I stood there and watched
the metallic horizon
tilt like a camera and fall.
And for just that second I could not lift my arms.
I was wearing an infinite invisible yoke.
It grew into my neck, pressed in on my throat.
Nothing could reach my head.
And I thought of his head, on all those pillows
the way he likes them, the way we fix them
away from his shoulders and neck.
As though he wears a yoke of air
only his head kept separate, high
everything else going under.

## Of Dresses, Colors, and 3:48 A.M.

The dress is still drying, the dress is still dye-ing, this formerly off-white silk brocade dress. It's lain overnight on two plastic chairs and it's kind of drippy, I'm a tad nervous; so far it's still the dark blue I want, but navy too often dries purple, or grey or tie-dyed. So 3:48 and I'm checking on that dress, adjusting the folds, shaking out the sleeves, flattening the hem and so far so good, so far still dark but then it's still pretty damp.
3:49 and suddenly I understand: Even if it does stay dark, as dark as now, it'll still be dry. And dry always means weak. It won't have that heaviness, that delicious substantial heaviness like those new-fangled fridge magnets or those lead shields when you get X-rays.
Yes, all of a sudden – 3:50 A.M. – this whole world seems too dry; it needs urethane, it needs a vaporizer. Like the floor after being washed, like skin from the shower, like ink from this pen, it all dries far too soon.
Only he in his hospital bed, water dripping through the J-tube into him all night every night; only he stays hydrated, only he stays irrigated safe and sound.
Yes, 3:51 A.M., I should put a J-tube in this dress, the seam
    maybe or zipper or hem;
I should sew a J-tube to the belly of this dress
to keep it basted
keep it juicy

keep it alive
keep it navy.

## Self Portrait With Catheter Bag #2

She is thinking about dying.
It gives her claustrophobia.
And she hopes, when it happens, she's tired.
She does a lot of things better tired.
Math. Scrabble. Sleep.
So maybe she'll die better, faster, easier.
Maybe she won't mind that space is disappearing
and what is taking its place.
Maybe she won't mind that time is collecting
and what it's collecting to.
She thinks about it a lot these days.
And oh, how she hopes she's good and tired.

## He Sleeps Raised

And I lie awake and stare. Not *at* him but *under*. All those pillows, sizes, shapes. Folded in half, folded in quarters. Over the mattress, under. And then gaps. Gaps and a tunnel. The cats run through it. Rats could also. It's a dragon's mouth, a broken puzzle. Or it's boards down the cellar, too many boards. Am I undersea or underground? Am I drowning tonight or already drowned?
I keep staring up at that concoction. I just lie awake and stare.

## Untitled

Even if we won the lottery we'd still have to wait five days for
    the check to clear
and two weeks to find a baby-sitter
six weeks to find a housekeeper
many months to put in a wheelchair lift.
As for celebrating at Le Bec Fin
it takes time to get a reservation
then it takes time to get served.
Oh, I'm sure the service is great.
But right now I'm so hungry
just so hungry.

## Temper Tantrum For That Taxi Driver

If God does everything, why doesn't he come down here and do this? Yeah, why doesn't God do toilet and why doesn't God do nights and I know God can create a stone so heavy he can't lift it but why doesn't he lift Jeff from that mattress?
Let him get his butt down here and wipe this butt, let him get off his ass and rub bedsore medicine into this ass. An eye for an eye, a tooth for a tooth, let God brush those back teeth, let him scratch just under that right eye. Also, God created arms, God created throats, let him range those arms, let him suction that throat. In general, God, get your shit down here and finish what you started.

## Writing As a Disability

If he can have chronic progressive incurable M.S., I can have
    chronic progressive incurable books.
Every time he needs another jar, I need another book.
Every time he needs a bedpan I need two new books.
And when he needs scratched
the top left part of the inside of his right nostril
or when something is caught between the two gold teeth
    bottom left back
or when the home health aide doesn't show
I need exacerbating books.

And when he calls "Mar"
I need a book signing.
"Dr. Marion Deutsche Cohen", I sign
or just plain "Marion", of maybe "Mar" in quotes.
In other words, it's not the books I need but the author.
Or the name of the author.
My chronic, progressive, incurable
exacerbating name.

## Demonstration: April 30,1992

Take-back-the-night, I want to take back midnight, the night's beginning, when you've almost fallen, almost landed, when you still know but don't know that you know, and I want back 2:30, that single point, the center of turning, sharp as novocaine and I want 3:30, another of the night's many wonderful middles, when you lie in a sphere, tucked into your childhood or your youth or your death, I want the night's middle and I want the night's endings, 4:00, 4:30, those pre-dawnings, pre-awakenings, when you've had enough but are taking more.

And 5:00, and 6:00, give me back my 6:00, and my 7:00, my 8:00, give me back my morning, give me back my day. Give me back my hours, my various hours, quit stalking me, quit jarring me, quit assaulting me, quit raping me; the night is mine, those hours are mine, I want them back, give them back.

## Bathroom Rumpus Again

Hillary Rodham Clinton doesn't do *this*.
And Hillary Rodham Clinton doesn't do *this*.
And this.
And this.
And this.
And this.
H.R.C. doesn't give keynote addresses about *this*.
H.R.C.'s father never made her do this.
H.R.C's secretary sent me a form letter answer to this.
Take this, H.R.C.
And this.

And this.
And this.
And this.

## Notes On Sleep Deprivation

When you do sleep you sleep fiercely. You condense your dream, or begin at the end.  Or you have two dreams at once.
You dream rapist-dreams, clutter-dreams, your laundry cart filled with furniture.
Or your floor has become a parking lot. You tremble with de-powerment.
Like your dream-time, your dream-space
is wrought with efficiency.
You court the rush, you crowd it all in. Space is in a hurry, too.

## Summer Exacerbations

He speaks with wind, takes deep breaths, or breaths that should be deep. Head held back, neck a trunk. And it's not poignant. Not right now. Rather, it comes out stern.
No, it's not a fuss, like the baby's cough. And not a fury, like the baby's cries.
No, it's not soft, not loving, not an individual but a type.
And stern.
That bears repeating. Stern.

## Summer Of '92

I am calling for help
but help isn't answering.
I call Community Care
get community doesn't care.
I call Family Services
get family disservices.
call Hospice
but don't prosp-ice.
call R.L.I.
rather sorrily.
I call articulately.
I call intelligently.
I call with dignity.
And they go u-huh.

Blue Cross won't cross.
Blue Shield won't shield.
And as for charities –
I don't need anyone to read to him.
I don't need anyone to sing to him.
And it's not his brow that needs to be wiped.

*continued...*

I keep calling help
and getting hell.
I keep dialing help
and getting on hold.
I keep yelling help
and getting u-huh.
I am calling for help
and getting hurt.

## Questions, 1993

Did they have social workers in concentration camps?
Did they talk about "intake" and "out-patient basis"?
Did their high-heels click as they walked down the halls?
Did they go into "the home" and "educate the family"?
Did they say "I understand" and "blame the system" and "u-huh"?
Did they hold orientation and stress-management workshops?
Did Blue Cross cover it?
Did they have Poets-in-the-Camps?
Did somebody get a grant?

## Progressive '93

He can still raise his arms.
can still turn his head
and keeps locating
miracle cures.
He stays insistently
on his diet
then goes insistently
off his diet.
He orders more stuff
from more catalogs
and wants me to wear
those pearls every day.
He wants everyone's number
in his Rolodex.
Even his enemies.
Even my friends.
This year's kittens
are on the third floor.
He hasn't seen this
year's kittens yet.
I should go to that room.
I should lie down beside.
I should write in that room.
I really should.

## More Notes On Sleep Deprivation

Not only do you dream hurriedly, you dream incorrectly. "I don't wish that," you say. "I don't fear that," "that's not my dream," and Freud agrees.

You try other dreams, that dream plus epsilon, that dream minus delta; a dream is a curve and you try both tangents and Freud shakes his head and shrugs.

You keep trying out all the various dreams; you go through the files, you go through the piles, and you say to Freud, "I have the interpretation; where is the dream?"

## Last Night's 2:00 A.M.

Instead of just plain "Mar"
he calls "Mar, are you there?"
Does he mean am I in the bathroom?
Or is somebody else on tonight?
Does he mean have I left him?
Or have I died?
At any rate, I like it
that he puts it that way
that he doesn't just assume
I'm there.

## Rehab

That tub they brought in, it's clean and blue
that same slippery too-blue blue
as that water-ride I just went through.
Maybe not skew
maybe not goo
but still, just waiting to receive my you.
He'll lie there surrounded by that crew
while their water sleezes anew
doing whatever they want it to.

## Reasons To Cry

So somebody can comfort you.
So somebody might comfort you.
So somebody should comfort you.
Also, same reasons as to laugh.

Laughing exercises the liver.
Crying exercises just behind the eyes.
And above the ears.
And those muscles all over
that shake
in that way.

## The Back Up Poem

*(He ordered four of those special air-mattresses, "as back-ups".)*

Back-up mattress.
Back-up pillow.
Back-up Ajax.
Back-up Brillo.
Back-up bedpan.
Back-up jar.
Back-up TV
and VCR.
Back-up shirts.
Back-up pants.
Back-up Panasonic.
Back-up Marantz.
Back-up plate.
Back-up cup.
Not to mention "Mar,
"can you come back up?"

Back-up waffles.
Back-up bananas.
Back-up books
on table manners.
Back-up smile.
Back-up frown.
Not to mention "Mar,
"can you come back down?"

## Thirty-Five Years

What if some serial killer decides, from now on, instead of
    spending his life killing many women
he'll spend his life killing one woman?
On the first date he begins.
On the second date he continues.
At the wedding he's halfway through.
Sometimes it hurts and sometimes it doesn't.
Maybe they have children
and they don't change his mind.
And all that time he has his friends.
And he meets them in bars.
"How's it comin' along?" they ask.
"Oh, it's comin' along," he answers.
"It's comin' along good".

## This Is a Home

*written on the occasion of interviewing
prospective home health aides*

This is a *home*.

This is not a hospital
not a school
not an office
not an organization.

And not an agency
in particular, not an employment agency.

And not a *group* home
not an *orphan* home
not a convalescent home
not a nursing home.

This is not my work address, this is my home address.
This is a home.
Isn't it? Is it?
This is a home, dammit, this is our home.

## Training New Aides: One Thing I'm Tired Of

Trying to make it look easy, so no huffing and puffing, not even breathing, just talking and lifting, nice and smooth, maybe even gesturing with one hand, maybe even gesturing with both hands, maybe even closing my eyes. Like, "I could do this blindfolded with my hands behind my back." Like, "I could do this and take care of a two-year-old and make breakfast at the same time." Like, "this isn't impossible," "this isn't ridiculous." What are we trying to sell?
What are we trying to buy?

## This Is a House

> *("Isn't is wonderful, how he keeps up the work on his solar collector?")*

This is a house.

Not a garage.
Not a factory.
Not a shipping yard.
Not a construction site.

Not an assembly line.
Not a machine shop.
Not a testing ground.
Not a stomping ground.

Nursing homes aren't set up for the solar and neither is this home.

This, I repeat, is a house
and a home
and I plan to keep it up.

## Self-Portrait With Catheter Bag #3

She is just standing there
not quite straight.
Just standing there
not quite curved.
Just standing there
as though by a lake
as though by a tomb
or as though on stage.

She has a friend who dabbles in stand-up comedy. Well,
*she* could do stand-up *tragedy*.
Not quite Shakespeare
(where there's a story line)
not quite a poetry reading
(where there's a poem line)
more like a tantrum
or the end of a tantrum
whereby some tooth is buck, some joint disjointed
some tail between some legs.

She is out of gas, out of oil
and has not changed her mind.
Whereby she just stands there
just hangs there.
To match the posture of the tubing
she just kind-of hangs.

## Significant Adolescent Dream

I've got my true love in bed with me.
Only something's wrong.
He's three inches tall.
Moreover, he dances like Rumpelstilskin.
Moreover, not in the center but in the far corner.
Moreover, he's connected to me by a cross between a string
　　and a pole.
I operate him as I would an artificial limb.

Not *terribly* wrong, mind you.
Just a bit of a damper.
He's still my true love.
And he can still talk.
"I love you," he says. "I need you."
The voice rattles more and more distant
and I clutch the remote control device
as adoringly as I would a telephone.

## Goofing Off As a Disability

*(for those who say "You need a break
every once in a while.")*

If he can have chronic progressive M.S., I can have chronic
　　progressive breaks.  If he can have daily M.S., I can have
　　daily breaks.
If he can have hourly M.S., I can have hourly breaks.
I need my breaks compounded continuously.

When he has M.S. a couple hours a week, that's
　　when I'll take a break a couple hours a week.
The day he stops having M.S., that's when I'll stop taking
　　breaks
give or take a few years.

## Ode To Able-Bodied-Ness

Moving! Ah, moving! I love to be moving.
Moving is grooving. Moving is soothing.
Drifting, shifting, lifting, sifting.
Dashing, flashing, thrashing, splashing.
Supercalifragilisticexpialidosis.
I do not have multiple sclerosis.

"Wild thing, I think you move me."
Wild thing, I think I move me.
Yes, put your briefs upon the shelf.
I'll do range-of-motion on myself.

I'm a shaker and a mover.
I'm efficient as a twofer.
Yes, I'm good at moving
and I'm improving.
So I think I'll move now.
What a good idea.
It's time for some movement
and I don't mean diarrhea.

I'll have a space race
a time climb.
I'm a vector collector
a tensor dispenser.

*continued...*

I embrace gravity
avidly.
I embrace magnetics
with extra credits.
I'm an action figure.
A *re*-action figure.
Yes, I'm big on action
and I'm gonna get bigger.

I'll move back. I'll move forth.
I'll move south. I'll move north.
I'll move to the country.
I'll move to the city.
I'll stay on the road.
I'll be moving pretty.
I'm addicted to moving.
I'm afflicted with moving.
Movers' Anonymous.
(movers autonomous.)
I'll move to Egypt
'cause I'm nulla-plegic.
I'll move to Brussels
and I'll take my muscles.
I'll move to Vancouver
and there I'll maneuver.
I'll make a movie.
I'll make my next move.

## Bedroom, Midnight

We lie on our backs
and stare straight up.
We see the ceiling, the ceiling alone
ethereal as a skylight
and full of centers.
Yes, here, now
it is vacuously true
that there is no respirator in this room
no wheelchair in this house
no tools, no metal
no papers on this floor.
And then the walls.
The upper walls.
This room is vacuously a vacuum.
Yes, the top half of this room
is free of our lives.
The top floats.
The top lifts.
This room is vacuously free.

## Progressive, Progressive, Progressive

He can still sniffle
still sneeze
can still turn his head
thirty degrees.

He still has the sexiest
lips in town.
He can still cuddle up
(well, cuddle down).

He can still get big
but not bold.
He can still have
but not hold.

It's begun, the era
of hospital stays.
In and out
more than two days.

The moon tonight
is so damn convex.
It doesn't shimmer.
It doesn't flex.

He's allergic to novocaine.
Tubes down his nose.
Arterial sticks.
His blood still flows.

Still, I do look pretty.
My cheeks are so red.
My hair is so fluffy.
I'm definitely not dead.

I'm his young wife, aren't I?
He can still call me kiddo.
Yes, I'm his young wife.
I'll be his young widow.

Ambition, these days
gives way to stillness
as disability
gives way to illness.

That moon hides behind
the curtain flowers.
That moon is the one
different flower.

*continued...*

I call the hospital.
They put him on.
It sounds like going.
It sounds like gone.

The cats regard each other.
The cats take posts.
The cats fill the room
like allover ghosts.

## Notes On Being Tired In General

1.
You feel self-conscious.
As though you're afraid you're gonna do something by mistake.
Fall on someone, pounce on someone.
It's as though you're coated, or novocained.
As though you've forgotten
the shortest route.

2.
Tired-in-general isn't the same as just-plain-tired. It's a state, a chronic state, chronic progressive incurable state. You learn-to-live-with-it, you-shall-overcome, and you don't fall, you don't pounce.

But it's not ordinary insomnia. No, it's not the habit of not-sleeping. You're not supposed to sleep. It's not the season for sleep.

No, the cure for tired-in-general is not sleep. The only cure for tired-in-general is sleep-in-general. Chronic, progressive, incurable sleep.

## Despair

Something doesn't want me.
Something has instructed the others not to want me.

It's not personal.
It was picked from a hat.

I should not feel hurt.
Only harmed.

## On the Train

I fear the next stop
as though the last stop were a job interview
or a job.

I fear the next day
as though the last day were my execution
which it is.

**Part II: Out Of the Frying Pan**

## The First Nursing Home Dream

It's admission day. We're in the office, all waiting around – he,
   his mother, father, me.
"Well," they ask, "who's the one we're admitting?"
And so tired am I that I forget.
I glance at his mother. "Hmm. She's sporting that worried look
   again. Try her." They do and it works, no more worried look.
Still, I glance at his father. Depression. Parkinson's. Not to
   mention worried look.
"Try him now." It works again.
I glance at the mirror by the door. Tired. Scared. Angry. Tired.
"Hey, don't forget me." It works with all of us. We fit right in.
Being taken care of becomes us all.
It becomes us very very well.

## The First Nursing Home Reality

Well, we've got two Congratulations, three Mazel Tov's, four Yays, and one serious "I'm really happy for you, Marion." First to say I'm sorry is a rotten egg.

## Not Grieving

They should have spouse-going-into-nursing-home cards. Not condolence cards, not sympathy cards, more like congratulations or thinking-of-you. I'd love to receive at least one of those cards. If not a medal, if not a paid professional position, if not a present, then at least a card.

## Sick

Bret gets sick, Elle gets sick, kitten gets sick, cat threatens sick.
I don't understand. I don't need to be reminded. I get the message, loud and clear:
Just because I've gotten rid of him
doesn't mean I've gotten rid of everybody.

## Sick #2

Yes, everyone gets sick.
As though they've all heard of my caregiving skills.
As though they think I'm looking for a new job.
But I fooled *them*.
I got sick, too
and told them I'm self-employed.

## Weepy These Days

Yesterday, watching Amadeus, I learned that Mozart was 34
    when he died. I had thought he was 37.
So now, 5:00 A.M., I lie awake, then *sit* awake
counting again
subtracting again
grieving for those three years.

## Welcoming Address To the Nursing Home Staff

I understand.
I see your problem.
You have a right to have a problem.
I know I shouldn't say I understand because I *don't* understand.
I understand.
You don't have to tell me.
Don't you dare tell me.
Tuff shit.
Shut up.
I don't understand.
This is a recording.
And one last word:
U-huh.

## The End Of That Dream

Yesterday Roberta said "I'm glad you finally put your foot
    down"
so last night's dream ended with my head embedded
in the softened ceiling.
I had slowly risen
happily flown
but, at the ceiling, had gotten stuck.
I could put my foot down
but not to the floor.

## Friend

Freda said you're a beautiful woman whose husband is dying
and it was as though she spoke each word slowly
as though she looked up, then down
and then back up
as though she asked permission
to speak each one.

## At His Mouth

There are four of them. Like the four seasons. Like the four directions.
There's the call-bell, the blow-tube, and two new sip-'n'-puffs.
Four mouthpieces, four microphones. They form a star, an almost-asterisk.
All those endpoints, like bugs around a lamp.
All those arrows, instead of a kiss.

## Following Him Into the MRI

I would not have followed him to the ends of the earth but I did go almost completely in there, head first, all the way to my waist. I had committed.

It was okay to kiss him, okay to keep fingers in his hair. I had brought a book, maybe a physics book, and maybe I read to him, read away that hour, or maybe we both then napped.

We just lay there, head to head, hand to hand, and there was light at the end of that very short tunnel, a huge waterfall of light.

## About Sex

The catheter gets in the way.
The J-tube gets in the way.
The diaper gets in the way.
And, once, shit got in the way.

Yes, shit happens.
Shit never stops happening.
There is never, in this biz
a season without shit.

## On the Toilet, Me

I flush first, wipe next.
Something soft and mushy taps the back of my hand.
Oh yeah, *my* shit.
What about
*my* shit?
I have shit
too.
I forgot about
my shit.

## Notes On a Current Pet Peeve

Green Bic pens. Remind me not to buy them. Green just isn't a dark enough color.
Green just isn't a strong enough flavor. Green is like yellow. Old wilt-y yellow. Yellow that's trying to get back to green.

I'm not blaming Bic; I'm blaming green. I'm also blaming his voice, that withering yellow-green voice. A voice that's trying to be navy-blue. A voice becoming transparent and white.

## Dream In Which I Was Only Talking

"I'm trying to make it so the people I love don't take away my life.
"People don't have the right to take away other people's lives.
"People who love each other don't take away each other's lives.
"I'm not gonna let the people who love me take away my life."

And then I said "What's the point of saying all this in a dream when I say it in real-life?"
But then I went on. "I guess dreaming you say something is different from merely saying it.
"Dreaming makes it a little more real."

## On the Need To Be Heard

Tears are transparent.
And their edges don't give them away.
Also, they're too small
to reflect anything much.
So you have to squint.
Or sob.
Or shake.
You can't just weep.
You have to cry.

## Dream Of the Dinner For Two

Tablecloth of cloth.
Silverware of silver.
And flowers. And candles.
And holding hands.

Why in the bathroom?
Because that's where all dinners wind up.
And why two toilets?
Because dinner for two leads
to twice as much shit.

## Where Loneliness Begins

My arms aren't empty, my arms are just fine, my arms have
  kids and cats and friends  to wrap like a present and tie like
  a bow.
It's my legs that concern me, my isolated legs, it's impolite to
  greet with your legs
and quite improper to hug with your legs.
Yes, loneliness begins where M.S. begins – the bottom, rock-
  bottom, away from what sees.
Where loneliness begins is where trees begin
close to the earth
far from the sky.

## Contemplating the Second Time Around

If I ever decide I want a true love in my life again
I might first have to go through strangers in my life.
Or my house.
Or my bed.
Or at least those sad and scary dinners
for two people who will be in love
but aren't
quite
yet.

## After a Bad Evening a Mean Little Voice Tries To Whip Me Into Shape

"You're not really alive, you know. You died in your sleep, or
 you died in your rest.
"Your alive days are over. You're dead and away.

"So whadder you hunting up recipes for?
"Whadder you picking up the phone for?
"Whadder you writing in your appointment book?
"And why are you staring at your child?"

"Well," I reply, "dead mothers stare at their children.
"Just like dead children stare at their mothers.
"Dead people can stare. Dead people may stare.
"Who says the dead don't stare?"

## The Fury Of the Living

A dying body is an area. A garden.
You sit on an edge, you get a side view.
And the garden has garden flowers.
"Please stay off the grass."

## Reading A Book This Particular Day

I am suddenly surprised that the paper isn't lined, or divided
 into squares. Each word needs to be in its own box.
All of a sudden the words are swaying, wandering off, getting
 lost. Oh, the letters hold tight; the letters make words.
But this page is threatened, this page is in danger.

This page needs gravity and magnetism.
This page needs suction tube and respirator.
This page needs range of motion.
This page needs something from me.

## The Misfortune Cookie #2

*(sequel to "The Misfortune Cookie" in Epsilon Country)*

Help! I'm being held prisoner at 2600 Belmont Avenue.
Help, I'm being beaten by a blow tube
molested by a feeding tube
raped by a suction tube
kidnapped by three wheelchairs converging in the hallway.
Help, I'm an
ambivalence slave.

It's Sunday again and I'm chained to this death
and from my life.
A whole family of professionals
cannot do this together.
I'm not really a prisoner any more.
But help, I have to keep reporting for parole.

**Christmas 1993**

Jesus couldn't move much.
He had many fixed points.
He couldn't draw up his knees
or wipe his nose
or make any other
minor adjustments.
Moreover, he was displayed.
He was 'way up there.

I hope that's not how it is for Jeff.
Lying there in that room, on that mattress
in between ranges-of-motion.
At least Jesus was vertical.
At least Jesus could flex.
At least Jesus could tap his fingers.
At least, for Jesus, it was only two days.

## August 3,1993

I forget that not all dying is drowning.
Some people breathe and see as they die.
And talk.
And move.
And toss and turn.
As people are dying
they're often also living.
I tend, these days
to forget about that.

## The Last Love Poem For Jeff

You are my you
My only you.
My Winnie the Pooh
My diddly doo.

Of all the animals in the zoo
I choose the ewe, I mean the you.
Of all the trees in Kalamazoo
I choose the yew, I mean the you.

Of all the letters old and new
I choose the u, I mean the you.
Of all the functions, f of u
I choose the identity, just plain you.

Ghosts say boo.  Cows say moo.
But who says you?
Only you.

## Progressive #Umpteen

He can still sniffle
still sneeze
still turn his head
twenty degrees.

He can't wriggle his fingers
can't make a fist
but on a good hour
he can pivot his wrist.

He can still use the (voice-
activated) phone.
Yes, he still has a voice
but it's monotone.

He can still sip.
Still puff.
Can still cough
but not enough.

He can still wonder
still worry
still remember
vegetable curry.

*continued...*

He fears death
even Heaven
but can still smile
when I mention Devin.

He has all his hair
all five senses
all three dimensions
all three tenses.

And why, these days
am I wanting to rhyme?
More than I used to?
More of the time?

Is it the same
as turning to humor?
A kind of hormone?
A kind of tumor?

And is it annoying?
Is it excessive?
Is it chronic?
Is it progressive?

## March 6, 1998

*(sequel to "December 29, 1989" in Epsilon Country)*

Maybe equations don't take care of themselves, maybe I have to keep checking on them
make sure the x's don't change into y's, make sure the epsilons don't change into deltas
make sure minus-signs don't keep poking their way in.
Even my new favorite equation, the one about F-bracket-x divided by the ideal generated by p of x, make sure that homomorphism still works, make sure the First Isomorphism Theorem doesn't become the Last Isomorphism Theorem.
And maybe the two sides of equations will become wings and carry them away. Maybe the equal sign will spin ninety degrees and become too tall, a barbed wire fence, block the two sides from each other, make it impossible to cross over.
Or maybe it'll all fly away, no such thing as math, math gets outside, gets physical, becomes physics, his physics.
I have to lift it, toilet it, wake up 2:00 AM to stretch its legs or scratch its nostrils, and I think I hear it calling Mar.

## Wanting To Rhyme

1.
Having to visit is bad enough
and being late is a sin
but worst of worst is having to write
*how* late, when you sign in.

2.
It's only once a week
and only 10:00 to 2:00
but while these hours are happening
it's like that's *all* I do.

3.
Chronic, chronic, chronic.
Progressive and progressive.
The latter I want more of.
The former I want less of.

4.
O Lord, let it be over
so we won't have to suffer.
He's suffered enough already
and I've suffered enough-er.

4.
Monthly Care Plan Meetings
include him, yessiree.
But we all raise our eyebrows
to a level he can't see.


5.
Every other second, now
it's suction tube time.
Don't anyone dare criticize
my rhythm or my rhyme.

## Courtship Memory

Outside my door
five minutes to day
we were kissing good-night
and I whispered "stay".

"Someday," I said
"some far-off day
"I'm going to change
"and want you away.

"I'll eat chicken satay
"and lemon sorbet.
"You'll be away
"and I'll want it that way."

It was misty and grey
the moon not a ray.
I continued to say
"hold me.
"Hold me against that day."

## Especially Progressive That Day

His voice, his ears
fading
paling.
Eyes drooping.
Head rolling.
"Jeff," I think, "wake up.
"You never really told me about yourself.
"Tell me, really tell me
"while you still have a voice and a mind."

## On Reading To Sick People

When you're reading they don't ask you to scratch just below
    the left nostril
or wipe the outside corners of both eyes
or range their lower right leg slowly twenty times.
The more you read the less they itch.
The more you read the less they ask.
Who was it? – Shaherazade? –
tale after tale
to hold off her enemies
distract her friends
escape her dying, her dead.

## Where I Stand These Days

There is a life
and I want it.

There is water
to drink.
There is food
to eat.
And there is air
to wave my arms in.

There are stores
to shop in.
Restaurants
to congregate in.
Bookstores, meetings, and conferences
to present at.

There is a book
my book.
There is a life
my life.

There is a life
and I have it.
I want to have it more.

## Signs Of Dementia

I should be thinking of lace, of doilies
the advantages of skeletons
branches without leaves

the usefulness of
the forgetful functor
the qualities of shadows
fatigue and sleep

I should be caressing this asymmetric snowflake, this two-leaf
    clover, this sieve of Aristophanes
should be quietly touching this delicate fractal
respectfully studying what's left.

## The Beginning Of Being Dead

I hope the beginning of being dead
is not like an amusement park.
I don't want to get swung, don't want to get whirled.
I'm afraid of forces, distances, afraid of losing the earth.
And I hope the beginning of being dead
isn't like the beginning of being alive.
I hope I don't have to get re-shaped.
I don't like spirals, don't like vortexes, don't like special effects.
And I hope the beginning of being dead
is only the *very* beginning.
I hope it doesn't last very long
very much.

## On Movies vs. Plays

I like movies better.
Plays are too close.
The actors can see and hear you
maybe play with you.
Someone can run into the middle of a play
can stop a play
can tear it down.
I like my entertainment passive.
I like to sit back in the dark
in the actors' future
in my own past.

## Chronic

He can still get a respirator
still get a J-tube
still get a trach
although it's all fake

still get antibiotics
still get a pic-line
still get blood gas
alas

go on Disability
go on Medicare
go on Medicaid
for another decade

still have a stroke
still have a coma
still get frozen
for another dozen.

There's always something else to do
and he wants them to.

## A Writer's Little Nightmare

My pen just ran out of ink.
So I pick up a pencil.
But the pencil also
has run out of something.

Any object can get tired
of being what it is.

## Thinking About the Second Time Around

How did I do it the first time around? All those lips, over all those streets, all either too wet or too dry, all pretending not to be lips. And then all those pants pretending not to be pants.
And all those lips and pants not being virgin this time, not the slightest possibility of virgin.
My lips, too. My pants, too. All those experienced lips and pants, all those not-his lips and pants, all those fishy little lips and pants.

## The Life and Habits Of the Well Spouse

I go through museums quickly. I pause only briefly, read the text briefly, "okay, okay, I get the idea."
Novels too. Math books, too. I might be the only one who skips to the end of a math book, "okay okay, I get the idea."

Everything is too chronic. Too much lingering. A deathbed that refuses to become death.   Too much too soon, too much too late, okay, okay, we get the idea.

## Deciding Against the Second Time Around

Alone doesn't have lips, alone doesn't have pants.
No one is still not him but at least I don't have to do anything
   with no one.

No one is better. Alone is better,
I'll take alone, thank you. I think I'll take alone.

## But the Dermatologist

He was so gentle with the novocaine. And he gave me assorted lotions.
Ten pretty bottles, all different colors.
And then he called in two other doctors.
They spent fifteen minutes deliberating about that two-bit mark on my back.
And he walked me over to the appointment desk and took five minutes to decide which number in March was two Tuesdays from now.
It felt like making a date.
I have to confess he's cute.

Pants? No.
Lips? No.
Beautiful? No.
But cute? Yes.

## A Mathematician In the Family

If the existence of none can imply the existence of many
if numbers so far can pair up to fractions so close
if equations of all sorts can create further lands and seas
but if complex can be the end of the story

then one thing can truly lead to another
other things can lead to still others
chronic can eventually turn acute

there can be death after life
perhaps there can be
an end to the story.

## The Second Time Around, More Thoughts and Fears

Lips are coated.
Saran Wrap. Urethane.
I don't want anyone breaking the seal.

Lips are packaged.
Lips are a blister.
Lips are their own country.

Lips have their own climate.
Lips are their own odor.
Lips are already a couple.
I don't need any more lips.

Lips have their own amniotic fluid.
It is not yet time to give birth.

## More About Lips

Especially when you're been sleeping
especially when you've been sick
then are lips especially coated.
then are lips especially private.

Lips are then to be respected.
Lips are not to be disturbed.
Lips, then, are brand new.
Lips, then, are a child.

## A New Vow

I will give you the best deathbed anybody ever had.

I won't French-kiss your drool
or have sex with your catheter.
But I'll scratch your scalp, wipe your nostrils, and adjust blow-
　　tubes to your heart's content.
I will love, honor, and (within reason) obey
for this very last time.

It can't be a *long* deathbed.
It's your last *hours* we're talking about.
No, I don't promise time.
I've run out of time.
I can promise only energy.
Instead of time
I promise energy.
Instead of chronic
I promise acute.

I'm not used to acute.
I'm a little rusty on acute.
I might have to wing acute.
Maybe I'm a little afraid of acute.
Still, I promise
my inexpert acute.

My half-baked, half-hearted, half-souled acute
as much as I can muster
'til death –
not much longer, please –
do
us part.

## Wanting Him To Die

Remember "Death Takes a Holiday?"
Well, it does.
(And paralysis and dementia do not.)
As traveling companions Death
has taken along the Law of Averages
the Laws of Probability
and the Laws of Cause and Effect.
Maybe the laws of exponents will go next.
Right on the day the syllabus says to teach them.
There I'll be, poised with my favorite
x-to-the-zero equals one, and the one will suddenly go blank.
One will have taken a holiday.
Zero will work triple-shift.

## Alone

When I leave the house in the morning cats can't lock me out,
    cats can't even follow me into the vestibule.
Cats can only stay behind the glass y-z plane
as I move further into the rain.

When I come home and ring the bell cats inside can't run to let
    me in, cats can only bounce around the first octant
buzz, shiver, sizzle, shriek
as I fumble inside my purse so bleak.

And if I fall asleep reading cats can only lie down beside me
sleeping with me in too much glare
in the lonely king-sized unit square.

## January 2001

I wear no wedding ring.
And I am not loved.
No one sings down the street for the love of me.
No one is thinking about me
right now.

## Online Personal Ads As a Disability

If he can have chronic progressive M.S., I can have chronic progressive online personal ads.
If he can have exacerbating unremitting incurable M.S., I can have exacerbating unremitting incurable personal ads.

Every time he needs another nose wipe, I put in another personal ad. Every time he needs another suction tube, I put in two personal ads.

At least I do them myself.
At least I don't ask for his help.

## Untitled

If it's none of it real, then the dream of math still means
    something, so does the dream of art. Music too, flowers too.
But what means the dream of love?
It means a mockery, it means an insult, it means a transparent
    smile.  Dreams are for one, love is for two
and the dream of love is nothing like love.
But still, still, I would like to dream of love, I mean a long
    dream, an ongoing dream, a realistic dream.
Life is but a dream so why can't I dream of love?

## Personals 101 (a series of limericks)

(My ad)
I'm vulnerable and I'm strong.
I'm pretty and witty and long.
All details below
explained by a pro.
No way you can figure it wrong.

"I'm ISO my last love."
Could that be Mariondove?
No, I'm afraid not
cause what he's got
is not what I'm in search of.

"Just Lunch" has been ever so kind
a few first-date no-no's to find.
Like past romance
and future plans –
in short, whate'ers on my mind.

Since he's paid Metrodate.com
there's no limit, how he can log on.
He can do a mass email
to every female
'til all of them are gone.

*continued...*

"Is anyone there?" they implore.
And hey, I'm there to the core.
But their biz is biz
and they're five-foot-six
and asking for five-foot-four.

At last! At last! At last!
A writer who writes – fantast!
and writes, and writes
and writes, and writes
the present into past.

ISO DEPTH AND GRACE.
It seems we've closed the case.
But what he means
is pleasant dreams
at his or at your place.

It's an absolute positive match.
So you write and he'll answer – natch?
You rant, rave, and rend
"Am I *sure* I clicked SEND?"
To keep sane, you send out a new batch.

## September 11 and the Single Woman

*"Men aren't asking women out any more."*

A state of war has been declared.
Not many men of my age-group enlist
but all have caught the fever.
They're reading about the war.
They're worried about the war.
They are not reading or worried about me.
Come on, fellas.
Have your hormones changed to war-mones?
Has love taken a holiday?
Are there no fish left in the sea?

## Hurt

The boys in grammar school didn't think of me that way.
The boys in high school didn't think of me that way.
Jeff no longer thinks of me that way.
But I *am* that way.
I am *so* that way.
I am, alas
so very much that way.

## March 22, 2002

The way a cat meows when she wants something she's not
    getting
the way she *keeps* meowing
not very loud
not quite in pain
not quite asking for help

that's the way I say "I hate you" to God.

I don't believe in God.
God doesn't believe in me.
Also, God sometimes beats me to the punch
or sneers "u-huh".

But I still keep it up.

Well, no matter what I say, *he* keeps doing.
So no matter what *he* does, I keep saying.
Just like that cat keeps meowing.
She has her meow.
It's the only meow she has.
I have my no.
It's the only no I have.

## Another No

Friends try to console me.
"*Everybody's* having trouble finding jobs."
"*Everybody's* having trouble finding love."
"It's been a bad year for *everybody*."

But I only sigh.
"Excuses, excuses….
"What excuse will
"the powers that be
"drum up
"next?"

## The Problem

What do associative arithmetics look like?
That is a question I ask.
It is not a question I am.

Must $m = 1$?
Must x-sub-r be prime?
These smaller questions
I also am not.

They are *in* my head.
*in* my bones.
*in* my heart, my eyes.

No, I have not become questions.
No, I have not.
I have not.

## Monday Morning, Unemployed

The rest of the world feels that cold sting.
The rest of the world sickens over breakfast.
To the rest of the world the powers whisper "You know darn well."

Unemployed on Monday feels like the dentist with novocaine.
You still feel something. And it's still Monday.

The rest of the world feels that cold sting.
And so do you.

## Perish

Not only is life a math problem
that I have to do.
Life is a math problem
that fate has already done *wrong*.

When a student gets a problem wrong
she believes me and fixes it.
But THIS is a bad student.
This student won't make it right.

I mark up the paper again and again.
And again and again it comes back wrong.
He is off by a factor of two
to some very large power.

Sometimes he lets me write in his notebook.
But he won't erase what *he* wrote.
He sends it off to a journal
and publishes it under my name.

## The Imposter

My life is evil.
It is pretending to be me.
It gets into my conversation, my CV, and my bank account.
It can do this because it occupies the same space and time as
    me
and because it is believed by most that you are what you live.
But my life is not me and I can prove it.
My life is indecisive and I am not.
My life is aging quickly and I am not.
My life has unresolved baggage and I do not.

My life is kidnapping me.
My life is suffocating me.
I must rescue myself
from my life.

## Conversation With the Mirror

Look.
Do not be ashamed to look.
What has been done to us
is not the same as what has been done *by* us.
My moving lips are not mocking you.
Your moving lips are not mocking me.
Do you remember, back in the 50's
our mother said "Never be embarrassed unless you did
    something wrong."
I know, I know, we are embarrassed anyway, but still, still
let us hold our heads high.
Let us stick together.
Let us look at each other.
Look.

## Self In 2001

*(with inspiration from Anne Sexton's "Self in 1954")*

I am not gullible.
I am only very open.
Open-minded and open-hearted.
I sit here sporting the look that caused him to say "you're
   lovely"
and does not cause him to say that any more.
I am not gullible.
I am only lovely.

I am also very pacifist.
Everything is too violent for me.
Even a flower
grows too quickly.
Even a bird
disturbs the air.
And the death penalty
is especially offensive this year.

As usual, I believe in wanting
or at any rate, I want.
Sometimes wanting feels like getting.
Other times wanting feels like needing.
All times wanting
gives me peace.

A toddler is told she is not allowed.
And she still keeps asking.
A child is told the odds.
And she says "but we might win".
A mathematician works on a problem.
She just keeps sitting there.
She can think of nothing to think but she sits there anyway.
I sit at the computer and search.
And then I search again.
Maybe it'll come up different this time.
Yes, sometimes the child of misfortune is gullible.
Optimistic.
Good at wishful thinking.
God helps those who help themselves
but this is not helping.
This is doing time.
This is doing energy.
And we might win.
We might win.

## How I Know I'm Still Alive

The ground still bears me up.
The sky still holds me down.
And the air between
still fits my lungs.
My hands hold flowers.
They do not slip down.
My friends still call me.
I'm allowed to go out and play.
Also, I'm getting older.
My cells are not stuck.
And Godiva's still sells chocolate
for me to eat in bed.

## How I Know This Is a Dream

What happens first is seldom cause.
What happens next is seldom effect.
It's all suspiciously spiritual.
And what happens next
is far too symbolic.
The things I say in dreams
make too much common-sense.
Moreover, I dream in color.
(At least I think it's color.)
And when I wake up
the colors do not change.

## How I Know About the Law Of Averages

Word of mouth.
And I read it in a book.
I hear it's very nice.
What a good idea.

## Parable Of the Life-Affirming Woman

It's kind of fun to affirm something that isn't there.
It's fun and it's possible.
Affirming isn't proving; there's no need for rigor.
For every epsilon there needn't be a delta.
There are many epsilon which, lacking delta
will take a one, a two-and-a-half.
Just any number.
Any number at all.

## A Short Song Of Agony

"I don't know what to do. I don't know what to do. What should
    I do?"
I know, I know: I'll do what I *have* to do.
But what should I do besides that?

## Short Agony #2

I'm so unhappy. I'm just so unhappy.
(And I shrug.)
I hate you, existence. And you hate me.
(I shrug again.)
(Then I shrug again.)
(How many shrugs do I have left?)

## Slowly

Jeff wanted me to range him slowly.
Now life wants to range me slowly.
I want life to hurry up.
I'm not the slowly type.

## A Bad Week

*To be is to be the value of a variable.*
*Quine*

There are too many variables.
I am some of them.

I am also too many values
of these too many variables.

I am both dependent and independent variables.
Maybe I'm also co-dependent variables.

True, I am not all of the variables.
There are variables that I am not.
But I stare at those variables
and wonder whether perhaps I should be.

I am too many functions.
Meaning, I am no function at all.
I would never pass the vertical line test.
Every spear pierces me
in too many points.

## Another Misfortune Cookie

*dream, 2001 — When one is sick / two need help.*
*Well Spouse Association slogan*

Help, I'm being held prisoner in a box.
The box is open on one end
but I am tied to the other.
Moreover, to this other end
is attached a second box.
Yes, every square is an edge
of exactly two cubes.
And now they are forcing me
to stand up tall and walk.
I must carry around two cages
not only the one I am in.

## Murphy's Laws Of Probability, 2001

1) Whatever can't go wrong will.

2) Whatever is least likely to happen to anybody else is most likely to happen to me.

3) The Law of Conservation of Opportunity: The more possibilities I find and cultivate, the least likely each is to occur.

4) (The flip-side of affirmative action) God hinders those who help themselves.

5) "To each according to your needs"
   and you don't have many needs.

6) "From each according to your capabilities"
   and you have many capabilities.

7) "God never gives you more than you can handle"
   and you're very good at handling.

8) The cluster of zeroes would have ended
   just after you gave up.

## Cochlear

If the medical profession were to offer an implant
–the Law of Averages
seven years' feast
citizenship
my life –
I'd accept the offer in a soul-beat.
I'd give up unlucky culture and go back to my roots.

I'd still be an unlucky sympathizer.
(Some of my best friends are unlucky.)
I'd march on Washington for unlucky liberation.
But I am not unlucky-identified.

Yes, when they went in there
when, past my skull, they came to that place
they would find that place so ready
so willing, so able.

They wouldn't have to do much.
The Law of Averages would slip right in there.
And when the anesthesia wore off
I would have no trouble adjusting.
I'd be politically incorrect.
I'd jump off the operating table
partake of the feast
happily average out.

## Roses

Along 20th Street, near Walnut, wishing for a man who would give me flowers when suddenly there they just were, lying in the street – the street, literally, about a foot from the curb. You couldn't miss them, they were a lamp of many bulbs, a coat of many colors, shades of red, yellow, orange, combo's, and brand spanking new, not a crease among them and all wrapped up in that clear triangular plastic.

And you know that Norman Rockwell drawing, cop stopping traffic so a mother cat can get her kitten safely across the street? Well, cars were slowing down, to avoid those roses, the drivers sporting the same smirk as Norman Rockwell's cop.

I wanted those roses for my new vase so I walked on over, there was another car approaching so just in case, I signaled, pointing down to those roses, I gestured, smiled, called out thanks as I rescued them for good.

Like a prom queen I carried them around. People stopped and complimented. A man had not given them to me but a whole community had, I carried them around like a baby, brought them home like bringing a new baby home, burst through the doorway and settled them in where they were admired and treasured by all.

## What's Theoretically Possible

A character in a dream can change the dream
if she's the dreamer.
A character in a story can change the story
if she's the writer.
*All* the characters in a play can change the play.
*None* of the characters in a movie can change the movie.
I mean, once it's taped.
And it is.

## Honorary

This week, there still being no man to give me things, the community came through once again, and not just temporary roses. This time 8th and Spruce presented me with just exactly the stainless top-o'-the-line dish drain I wanted, it's pretty, not only practical and then 21st and Spruce awarded me this really cool white wastebasket.
Maybe eventually the community will give me a job or a man. Something that is something. Something in my class.

## Cancer Scare

No, I absolutely definitely cannot live as a dying person (I mean more dying than before). I cannot live with no future (I mean less future than before). I cannot live knowing that everything I do is for those I leave behind, and that only today counts and not tomorrow

cannot live knowing that I am only pretending to live, knowing that even if all this has been real, it won't be for much longer, cannot live with things this unreal, knowing I tried, I really did try, but it's only a dream after all.

## Mozart To The Gills

As I play him I talk to him, pretty cozily. "Oh," I quip, "you're just soooo mischievous."
At a particularly mischievous passage I call out, "Now, that's *bad*. That's very very naughty."
And when I get it right, "Yes!" I exclaim. "Yes!"
By the end, though, I feel that rumbling behind my cheeks then a wetness on my chin.
Because of what Mozart is mischievous *against*.

## The Beginning Of Courage

I'm getting used to this already, having a year instead of twenty, mini-future instead of maxi-future, being a temporary human being (more temporary than before).
In my usual style I have survived this, and quickly. I can do this, I can live this way

And now to the practicalities: A temporary human being does not need to go to Singles Events. A temporary human being does not need to find a tenured position, a temporary human being does not need to start another book or do more house renovations.

A temporary human being does need to keep on being a teacher to students, a friend to friends, a mother to children. A temporary human being does need to keep on being the best being she can be.

A temporary human being has less future to worry about but more present.

## Diarist's Strike

There's a new online review of my book.
I had another job interview.
I presented math poetry at Bridges conference.  One of my
   colleagues there offered me a job  and a man (both long
   distance).
My back pain means scoliosis and osteoporosis.
I don't have cancer.

But I refuse to hit that notebook.
I refuse to repeat the maybes.  I refuse to repeat the no's.

"Oh, she's upstairs writing in her diary," said my mother.
"There she goes, writing in her diary," said my father.
"Oh boy, let's see what she's gonna write in her diary," say the
   powers
then, rubbing their hands together, "and let's see what we can
   do about it."

Yes, the powers read my diary.
They do not read my email.
They do not read my lips.
They do not read my poems.

## Another Helpful Metaphor

Spring comes late most years.
I can pretend it's spring I'm waiting for.
I can pretend I'm waiting
for something that will come.
I can pretend I'm waiting for the same thing
as everybody else.

## I Disguise My House

Change the stucco to smooth.
The stairglide to stairs.

Flatten out the stove.
Fluff up the pillows.

Bleach the walls.
Darken the floors.

Cover the air-conditioner.
Un-cover the back wall.

So the powers will look for me
in some other house.

## "Memento"

I have no trouble with short-term memory.
But the powers do.
Yes, the powers keep forgetting
what I've done lately.

Ah, but *long*-term memory.
The powers have plenty of that.
*I* might not remember
the boys-in-high-school
how they dubbed me Stretch, Math Brain, Marion Dutch
everything but somebody to love.
And *I* might not be fixated on my father
mimicking the way I said "benk"
and never sending me off to school or Y dances
with arm-length adorations.
I let bygones be bygones.
But the powers remember
bygones well.

Yes, they know my history
(obstetric and otherwise).
And they keep to the tradition
keep to the old ways.

Yes, they're very good at old times.
Not very good at the new.

## The Revolt Of the Chosen

I reach out my arms
at first horizontally, then obliquely
finally out to the sky.

I am begging to be human.
Begging to be awake.
Begging to be real
before I die.

O, Law of Averages!
Why hast thou forsaken me?

Keep in mind that the Chosen Ones
have *not* chosen
have only *been* chosen.
And we are demanding
to be un-chosen.

It is time to be civilians.
Time to be citizens.
Time to be the Choosing Ones.
High and mighty time.

# Part III: Out Of the Fire

## Falling In Love

Like any learner I am slow.
No matter how long before I say something
there is a pause before it is true.

Like any learner I am afraid.
Points are blinking, lines are shimmering
and I cannot yet touch.

Like any learner I am stupid.

Like any learner I am ignorant.

Like any mathematician I have to sleep on it.
Go through my days, my weeks on it.
I cannot be given.
I must first prove.

Like any neighborhood this is not a point.
It's bigger than epsilon
bigger than delta
bigger, even, than one.

## Songs For the Good New Year

Before I can sing happy songs
I have to un-sing the sad songs.
To the listener un-singing sounds like singing.
But inside the singer un-singing is like un-doing.
"When you're dying your whole life passes before your eyes."
But you are not living that life.
You are un-living that life.
Maybe, when you're being born, your whole death passes
    before your eyes.
And yes, you are un-dying that death.
You are working very hard.

## Lips and Pants

are very much okay.

## Dream Of Hanky Panky

It's bad enough, that recurring dream of Jeff taking a week off from the nursing home to pay a surprise visit. What do I need the new expanded version for, where upon his arrival my new love is napping in the bedroom?
And why does Jeff hafta decide he needs a nap, too?
And I've seen enough horror movies, why would I need his paralyzed hand on the doorknob – slow, menacing, almost there?
–- "No! No! You can't go in there!"
"Why not?"
"Because ... because ... you just can't ..."
"But why not?"
"We ... we ... we hafta go shopping."

Well, we do.
We really do.

## My New Love In the Early Morning

He stirs (not spasms)
all by himself.
He turns over
all by himself.
He puts his arms around me
all by himself.

## A Quiet Man

A quiet man doesn't go into details.
A quiet man doesn't sing down the streets for the love of me.
But a quiet man buys me chocolate.
A quiet man has a database of the books I want.
When I leave the house in the morning, a quiet man runs downstairs to lock me out.
When I fall asleep reading, a quiet man turns out the light.
And a quiet man is thinking about me right now.

## Dream Of Someone Dying

He lies wounded in the street.
I call for an ambulance but they send a car.
"You called for a writer?"
"Writer?! No, I called for a doctor."
"Oh, well, sorry. I'm a writer."
"Huh? Why'd they send a writer? I don't need a writer. *I'm* a writer."

I called for a doctor but got a writer.
I got something that I already am.

## Progressive Becomes Progress

He can still see
still hear
and *we* can hear *him*
if we draw near.

He can still hear
still see
and still has that same
very long CV.

He can still feel pain
but not pleasure.
His blood still flows
but at half the pressure.

His heart still beats
but twice as fast.
His flag still flies
but at half-mast.

He can still nod yes
and roll his eyes no.
He can still let on
but he can't let go.

Yes, though it's not
so cost-effective

he holds to that
Advance Directive.

His leg is thick.
So is his arm.
But he still displays
that particular charm.

Yes, he gives the facade
of rationale
so still would pass
a psych-eval

so he can still
change his will.

## One Woman Show

I, the one he began with and the one he'll end with
am acting out this deathbed scene.
I pretend to say "Hey, I just took Devin to visit USP. Yeah, I've
    been taking him to visit the various colleges. Yesterday we
    went –" And then I pretend to pause.
And then I pretend to ask, "Do you want me to talk about this
    kind of thing?" And when he nods, I pretend to continue,
    yesterday's Temple, tomorrow's Drexel.
And then I pretend to fall quiet. I pretend to hold his hand.
I pretend to be the only one not bustling about
just being there, the one he began with, the one he'll end with
the one who's been too much in the middle.

## The Jeff Complex

Everyone has the Steve Hawking complex; nobody has the Jane Hawking complex.
And everyone has the Jeff complex; nobody has the Marion complex.
There they congregate, there they pace. There they brood, there they pray.

Everyone's pacing and praying for Jeff; no one's pacing and praying for Marion.
"What a will to live", they go, not "what a wimp to die".

No one talks about Marion's will to live (I mean live a *life*)
everyone knows what to make of Marion
everyone can stay away from Marion
Marion's a boring healthy deal.

## Instead Of Dying

Instead of dying he's getting transferred.
Instead of dying he's getting a new ventilator.
And there's a special meeting.
Instead of dying he calls more meetings.

Instead of dying he wants more heroics.
He's quite the hero; I'm quite the villain.
Instead of dying he's getting more living.
I thought this was it but it's only another this.

## This Versus It

*"I hope this is it."*

If *this* this isn't it, then the *next* this better be it.
I hope there aren't too many this's before we get to the it.
How many this's can a soul take?
Of course, the it will probably also be another this.
But it'll be a short this.
Maybe a sweet this.
A this destined
to become a that.

## Death Still Takes a Holiday

The Law of Averages is back on the job.
Cause and Effect are back on the job.
Even the job market is back on the job.
But death is still AWOL.

The doctors are going crazy.
The nurses are going crazy.
The insurance company is going crazy.
And the kids and I ...

well, acceptance is what we're crazy with.
Chronic acceptance. Progressive acceptance. Incurable,
    exacerbating acceptance.
That's what we'll all die of.
The fifth stage of grief.
The stage that's here to stay.

## Like a False Pregnancy

*(dream material)*

The kids phone me, one by one. "We talked to the doctor and he told us Dad *isn't* dying."
His brothers, too. My sister, too.
And the hospital. "How dare you put words in our mouths?"
And the funeral home. "Whadder you wasting our time for?"
And Jeff. "Reports of my fatal illness have been greatly exaggerated."
And my therapist. "Now, I can see why you'd indulge in a little wishful thinking. But this is ridiculous."

## One Line Untitled

We said *quality* of life, not *quantity* of life.

## Phone Call From the Hospital A La Molly Bloom

*October 12, 2003*

*Yes*
Yessie yessie yes
calling-Roz-yes
calling-Cathy-yes
calling-Norma-yes
calling-Freda-yes
emailing Well Spouse friends yes
emailing the Separation / Divorce group yes
emailing work and getting a week off yes
funeral yes
home memorial yes
Inglis House memorial yes
USP poetry reading memorial yes
my own particular eulogy in which I also eulogize the kids and
  me yes

no more toilet, no more lift
no more nights and no nightshift
no more J-tube, no more suction
Life's just chicken soup and lukchen
(Yes, today, yes tomorrow, yes forever by induction)

*continued...*

No no no,
H.M.O.
Yes, yes, yes,
TIAA CREF.
Yessiree, yessirah.
Yessiray, la de dah.
Seeya later, respirator.
After 'while, pressure dial.
Take your share, Medicare.
Take the shade, Medicaid.

*Yes!* under my breath.
*Yes!* behind my back.
But still, that was a *yes*.
Take that for a *yes*.

## On Getting Engaged the Day After My Husband Dies

*October 13, 2003*

If the Good Lord disapproved of opposite extremes, he
   wouldn't keep making them happen.

He wouldn't make bad mail arrive on Saturday.
He wouldn't make people die on their birthdays.
And he wouldn't make a woman, nine months pregnant, give
   death instead of birth.

If he can dish it out, he can take it.
And you should see the ring. It's so pretty.

## Calling a Spade a Spade

*October 14, 2003*

Because I might have regrets
and because he was so unwilling to die
I lift up the spade
fill it with dirt
and gently trickle it over.

The spade is heavy.
The dirt is heavy.
But not as heavy as *he* was
during those six years.

I lift again.
But not again.
And not as high.
And not onto the toilet.

And not in the middle of the night.

## Love Poem For a New Love

O will you be my you?
Can I look deep into
your eyes – I mean your pu-
pils, all the way down to
your brain, the heart of you?

And can I stay awhile?
Perhaps not near but far?
And can I know securely
the you I think you are?

Jeff used to be my you.
But now I want you to.
Yes, can the you be you?
Can I be your you, too?

And when you say I do
will you mean I or you?
I can't be my own you.
And so I need you to.

Tonight I can't help thinking
what the Nazis used to do
and so I need my you.
And that means I need you.

*continued...*

I can't stop being me
and so I need a you.
O please remain my you.
Don't pull a switcheroo.

## Wedding Preparations Former Well Spouse Style

If he could have chronic progressive MS, I can have chronic progressive white lace.
If he could have exacerbating MS, I can have exacerbating vintage silk flowers.
If he could have multiple sclerosis, I can have multiple wedding dresses.

And if he could lead a life too long and too full of heroics
I can have a wedding like that, too.

At least white lace and flowers don't keep anybody up at night.
Or maybe they do.
At least it's only for this summer.
Or maybe it's not.

## Wedding Vows

I have said that I don't think of weddings in terms of vows (only celebration).
Still, I hereby vow that, on this our wedding day, I will look at you often.
And I will stay by your side.
I vow that, if I am not already there, you will turn around and find me close by.
I will forget about the white lace and flowers and be only with you.
And you know how, after the ceremony, they say "You may kiss the bride"?
Well, why can't the bride and groom kiss during the ceremony?
I promise to do all of it.
All day.

Of course I will love you as long as it is possible to love.
Of course I will never hurt you unless dementia forces me to.
Of course, if not obey, I will love and honor you 'til death do us part  or 'til life do us part.
But this vow is not about the rest of our lives.  It is about today our wedding day.
I will love and honor and even obey you
today.

## Impossible Dreams

I would like to be, for you, something that doesn't come to pass
something more than flowers or trees
something more in the line of a theorem.

It's not my fault that even I shall come to pass.
If I had a choice, I would *not* come to pass.
If I had a choice, I would be a theorem.

I would like you to look at me as though you believe that I won't come to pass
and then I could look at you as though to say you're right.
I am the main theorem.
I might split up into many cases
but I will always be true.

## Post

Post-polio doesn't concern me because I never had polio.
What concerns me is post-well-spouse.
Post nights, lifting, and toilet.
Post wheelchairs every day.
Post so many silly questions that I run out of silly answers.

I could never again be that many variables.
I could never again have that many capabilities.
I could never again want that furiously.
I could never again shrug that many times.

## Dream That Jon Acquires a Wheelchair

Some stranger gives it to him.
And he's happy to accept it.
Immediately he sits down and asks to be wheeled around.
And then he slumps, body and head, and sports that
    expression-less expression.
"Jon," I command, "get outa that wheelchair this instant".
But he doesn't.

## The Human Spirit

(1)
A roach is a hole, a tiny traveling hole, an off-place where the floor is not a floor, the table not a table, the very house no longer ours.
But as the hole moves along, the floor comes instantly back.
Yes, how readily we reclaim our territories.
And how healthy, that the hole leaves no path. How nice, that where the roach has been is not discolored
that although every spot is where some roach has been, we continue to use it, and use it well.
With but a wipe now and then we keep living in our houses
eating off our tables, standing on our floors
thinking of them as solid
and not full of holes.

(2)
A cat is a hole, a soft hole, a warm hole, a hole to come upon,
   a hole to sit down with.
A cat is a hole in our dead matter. All of a sudden the rug, or
   the chair, breathes.
All of a sudden the bed, or part of it, beats.
All of a sudden something turns over and wants to be pet.
And yes, everywhere is where some cat has been, or will be
and there is, everywhere, that settling, those pulsings.
Everything, if you look close and long enough, has the
   firmness and the friendliness of a cat.

## Dream Of Easier Changes

I am lost, lost at night.
But it is not very dark.
And the street looks familiar.
Also, I have not lost my purse
merely left it home.
Nor have I lost Jon
merely left him home.
Moreover, I am holding a pen
and I have been using it.
True, I have been writing on no paper
but this is the kind of lost
where I know I'll soon be found.

## Possibilities

When creatures in movies about advanced galaxies get shot or knifed, it's not a problem. The wound quickly closes, leaving no scar.
And we in the audience say that's magic, can't really be.
But when our creatures get shot or knifed, our screams soon switch to sobs.
It still hurts but not as much.
Even in our galaxy, there's enough healing, and enough magic
for that.

## Notes

– Although I believe that the poems stand on their own (as many of them have in the journals in which they first appeared), I also believe that the explanations given here will enhance their meaning. It is in that spirit that I offer them:

P. 22: A J-tube is a particular kind of feeding tube. At the time of that poem's writing, Jeff needed to use it only for liquids.

p. 27: "Suction that throat": Because Jeff's throat was partially paralyzed, and partially numb, he didn't swallow properly and stuff collected in his throat and lungs. There was a suction tube right near his bed, and he would need to have somebody suction him pretty often.

p. 29: "Nights" refers to the fact that, because Jeff was paralyzed, he could not take care of even his simplest needs, such as itch-scratching and turning over. So he would wake me up many times during the night.

"Quit jarring me" refers to the fact that, when he had to go to the bathroom #1, we would use a jar. At night we kept several jars by his bedside.

p. 30: Many will recall how Hillary and Bill, in particular Hillary, tried to work towards adequate health care in this country. However, I knew that she had not experienced what I had experienced (in particular, not "nights, lifting, and toilet"), nor would her concentration be on "custodial care". I knew that, even if her goals were to be reached, that would do little for well spouses. That poem expresses my bitterness about that, as well as my anger and anguish over "toilet".

"H.R.C.'s father never made her do THIS" refers to the fact that her father had been ill, but had died rather quickly so was not *chronically* ill. Thus she wasn't a caregiver for very long.

p. 33: R.L.I. is the acronym for Resources for Living Independently, one of the several resources for situations like ours. However, most of what they offered, in our own experience, seemed to be mostly for show. In particular, they would give us lists of home health aides, and everybody on all of those lists, without exception, either didn't "do that kind of work any more" or turned out, very early on, to be unreliable. It is indeed very difficult to find home health aides who can handle people who are completely paralyzed ("dead weight"); however, even taking that into consideration, R.L.I. was inadequate in that respect.

p. 36: Jeff tried many alternative diets, in an effort to cure himself. However, as each diet turned out not to be a cure, he would abandon it – sometimes *before* this was apparent, possibly to avoid facing up to the fact that it would not work. In general, he desperately, and understandably, clutched at straws.

p. 39: He had to *be* bathed because he couldn't move.

p. 45: "work on his solar collector" – Jeff invented a new type of solar collector, which received a lot of newspaper publicity, but he was unable to find a distributor to even make a working model. He and friends would ineffectually set up shop in our living room.

p. 70: "call bell", etc.: He couldn't move but he could still breathe, so there were devices which helped him call "the desk", turn on the TV, use the phone, and so on.

p. 78: "where M.S. begins" – Often paralysis hits the legs first.

p. 82: "range of motion" – Somebody else had to move his limbs, in order that they not atrophy.

p. 83: This poem is about visiting days – basically I didn't particularly enjoy them.

p. 86: "the you" – In my book "Epsilon Country" there are two love poems beginning "You are my you".

p. 88: Devin is our youngest son. At the time that Jeff went to live in the nursing home, Devin was almost eight years old.

p. 89: Jeff was a physicist, and a very prominent one.

p. 95: "a book / my book" – "Dirty Details: The Days and Nights of a Well Spouse" had just been published (Temple University Press).

p. 96: "forgetful functor" – something in math (category theory); it's an operator that tells you to "forget" a particular structure on a set.

"sieve of Aristophanes" – Take all the integers, remove all the multiples of 2, then of 3, then of 5.... What's left are the prime numbers.

"fractal" – another math concept; the shape is very intricate.

p. 105: "complex can be the end of the story" – All reasonable equations have at least one complex number as a solution; thus we don't need to define more numbers in order to solve equations.

p. 110: "Death Takes A Holiday" is a movie.

p. 121: In a caregiver's life so many problems and questions arise that she is forced to constantly "bother" people in charge. I used to say to them, "It's not that I *am* a problem; it's that I *have* a problem." I often felt that I wasn't believed.

p. 131: "for every epsilon there needn't be a delta" – the opposite of the definition of continuity, in calculus.

p. 134: "range" – the verb corresponding to "range of motion"

p. 138: There are Cochlear implants for deaf people, to make them hearing. The deaf community has issues around them;

many don't want to give up their deaf culture.

p.153: "Points are blinking, lines are shimmering" – a recurrent line, and theme, in "Crossing the Equal Sign", my book of poems about the experience of mathematics (Plain View Press)

p. 161: "Advance Directive" is a legal document which an individual can have drawn up; it dictates what should be done when one has a terminal illness. Jeff's advance directive stated that all heroics be performed, to keep him alive as long as possible; this made life very very difficult for his family as well as for the nurses and doctors.

p. 163: Steven Hawking is a well-known physicist who has lived for close to fifty years with A.L.S. (a progressive disease which, like multiple sclerosis, involves paralysis). He has become a huge legend in his own time. Jane Hawking was his wife for many decades, until they divorced.

p. 169: Of this collection, this is the poem that I most hesitated to put in, knowing all the while that I must. I realize that to some it might sound harsh and uncompassionate towards Jeff. I hope that the previous poems convey how relieved I was, for all concerned; not only would he not suffer, not only would I no longer have to worry about further financial insecurity and abuse, but closure was now possible for our children, and for the family as a whole. I worry that those (grown) children might now feel upset by reading this poem, but I also feel that the story would be incomplete without it. Relief to the point of ecstasy was indeed my first and main emotion at the time. I had already, for over two decades, felt compassionate for and fond remembrances of Jeff, and it had already, many times over, been time for him to die.

The Well Spouse Association is an association of and for well spouses, meaning those who are spouses of chronically ill or disabled people.

The Separation/Divorce Group was a group which I belonged to and helped found, consisting of well spouses who were considering separation or divorce.

Inglis House was the name of the nursing home where Jeff lived for the last ten years of his life.

USP (University of the Sciences in Philadelphia) is where I was teaching at the time.

TIAA-CREF is a pension plan for teachers.

## About the Author

Marion Deutsche Cohen has published a total of nineteen books, among them *Crossing the Equal Sign*, poetry about the experience of mathematics, also published by Plain View Press. Among her other books are *Dirty Details: The Days and Nights Of a Well Spouse* (Temple University Press, PA), *Surviving the Alphabet* (Huge Pathetic Force, PA), and *Epsilon Country* (Center for Thanatology Research, NY). She teaches math at Arcadia University in Glenside, PA, and 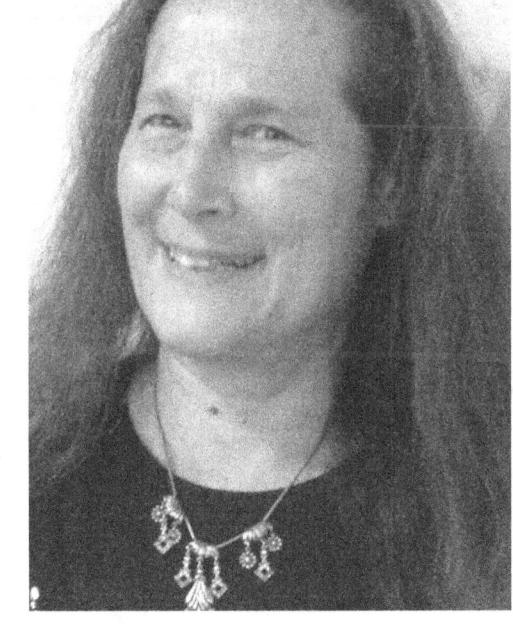 received her math Ph.D. from Wesleyan University in Middletown, Connecticut.
In l977 her first husband was diagnosed with multiple sclerosis, during the same season that their third baby died at the age of two days. The couple went on to have two more children (living), and for 24 years Marion was a loyal

and loving well spouse. When the illness began to involve dementia, and Jeff became verbally abusive, Marion left the marriage, eventually finding new love. That 26-year odyssey is what this present book is about.

She has been known in both the bereaved parent and the well spouse communities for her books and other writings. In particular, The Well Spouse Association (www.wellspouse.org) has been very helpful to and supportive of her. Other interests have been classical piano, singing, Scrabble, thrift-shopping, home-schooling, and spending quality and quantity time with her four living children, two grandchildren and a third on the way, two cats, and Jon.

www.ingramcontent.com/pod-product-compliance
Lightning Source LLC
Chambersburg PA
CBHW052029070526
44584CB00016B/1966